NUTRITIONAL HEALING

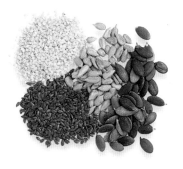

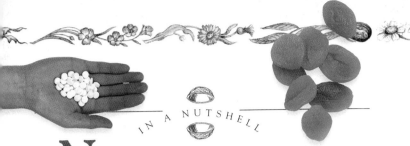

IN A NUTSHELL

NUTRITIONAL HEALING
A STEP-BY-STEP GUIDE

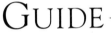

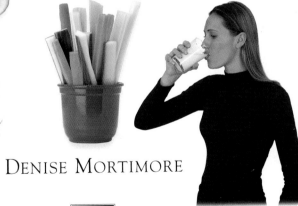

DENISE MORTIMORE

ELEMENT

SHAFTESBURY, DORSET • BOSTON, MASSACHUSETTS • MELBOURNE, VICTORIA

© Element Books Limited 1998

First published in
Great Britain in 1998 by
ELEMENT BOOKS LIMITED
Shaftesbury, Dorset, SP7 8BP

Published in the USA in 1998 by
ELEMENT BOOKS INC
160 North Washington Street, Boston
MA 02114

Published in Australia in 1998 by
ELEMENT BOOKS LIMITED
and distributed by Penguin Australia Ltd.
487 Maroondah Highway, Ringwood,
Victoria 3134

NOTE FROM THE PUBLISHER
Any information given in this book is
not intended to be taken as a replacement
for medical advice. Any person with a
condition requiring medical attention
should consult a qualified practitioner
or therapist.

Designed and created with
The Bridgewater Book Company Ltd

ELEMENT BOOKS LIMITED
Creative Director Ed Day
Managing Editor Miranda Spicer
Project Editor Katie Worrall
Production Manager Susan Sutterby
Production Controller Sarah Golden

THE BRIDGEWATER BOOK COMPANY
Art Director Terry Jeavons
Designers Kevin Knight, Jane Lanaway
Managing Editor Anne Townley
Project Editor Julia Roles
Photography Ian Parsons
Picture Research Vanessa Fletcher
Scientific Illustrations Michael Courtney
Three-dimensional Models Mark Jamieson

Printed and bound in Great Britain

British Library Cataloguing in
Publication data available

Library of Congress Cataloging
in Publication data available

ISBN 1-86204-245-4

The publishers wish to thank the
following for the use of pictures:
Hutchinson: pp 6TL, 7T,
16B, 17; Image Bank:
p 21B; Science Photo
Library: pp 10, 28; ZEFA:
pp 6R, 13, 39B, 40, 52TL

Thanks to: Aje Jikiemi-
Roberts, Elin Osmond,
Donna Poplett, and Andrew
Stemp for help with photography,
and to Felicity Jackson for freelance
project management

Contents

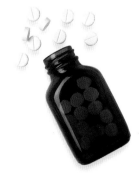

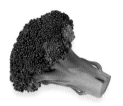

What is nutritional healing?

NUTRITIONAL HEALING IS *the practice of using a wide variety of wholesome foods and nutritional supplements to improve health and prevent disease. It is a very practical way of overcoming illness and promoting health naturally, without the use of toxic drugs. The diets are very straightforward and anyone can partake in this system of healing.*

LEFT *Each person has a unique body chemistry.*

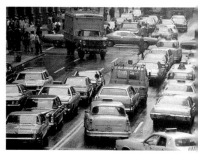

ABOVE *Pollutants from heavy traffic can damage the body's ability to absorb nutrients.*

With nutritional healing, the body is encouraged to heal itself by proper nourishment of the tissues and organs where disease has originated. Furthermore, it heals the whole body, not merely removes symptoms, strengthening it to resist disease.

As with all reputable therapies, the holistic and individual approach is vital. Since each person has a body chemistry which is unique to them (arising from genetic inheritance, constitution, lifestyle, and environment), each individual needs a nutritional program to suit their own particular needs.

The human body is extremely complex and has very specific requirements for good health. Apart from the essentials such as oxygen, water, warmth, shelter, and sunlight, the most important factor is optimum nutrients – proteins, carbohydrates, fats, vitamins, and minerals.

Unlike the immediate reaction from oxygen deprivation, for example, a deficiency in essential "food" nutrients can result in anything from mild, almost imperceptible ill health, through a wide range of symptoms, to the slow development of chronic conditions which rob us of the quality of life. Environmental pollutants, and the use of antibiotics and other drugs also cause changes in the body, often affecting its ability to absorb nutrients, and preventing elimination

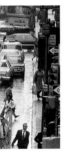

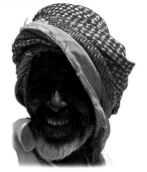

ABOVE *Each person needs a nutritional program to suit their specific needs.*

of toxins. Add an unhealthy lifestyle, and the body starts to develop a toxic load which will eventually lead to disease.

Fortunately, the body has a powerful self-healing capacity, if encouraged with the proper use of food and nutritional supplements, and a little tender loving care.

AN UNHEALTHY LIFESTYLE

The effects of poor nutrition will be increased if the body is further compromised by an unhealthy lifestyle that includes:

- insufficient exercise
- smoking
- high stress levels
- lack of proper rest
- lack of relaxation

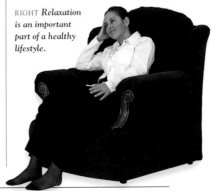

RIGHT *Relaxation is an important part of a healthy lifestyle.*

A short history

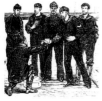

ABOVE *Sailors used to suffer from scurvy due to a lack of vitamin C.*

IN THE WEST *the diet has changed in an unprecedented way, so that people are now eating foods quite different from their evolutionary requirements. Modern living also brings with it additives and pollutants in food, air, and water. In addition, it produces toxic chemicals from our own over-stressed metabolism. All these substances are "foreign" materials which our bodies cannot recognize. They put a great demand on our digestion and metabolism, since they have to be rendered harmless and eliminated.*

They also increase our requirement for essential nutrients, the substances necessary for growth, normal functioning, and maintaining life. Nutrition is the name given to the processes involved in taking in nutrients from food, absorbing them efficiently, and utilizing them appropriately. Essential food nutrients must be supplied by our dietary intake because they cannot be made by the body.

Single nutrient deficiencies tend to be rare but multiple deficiencies often occur, particularly in those people who are already unwell. Multiple deficiencies are also common in individuals consuming a typical Western diet, which is characterized by many excesses and "essential-nutrient starvation," leading to biochemical chaos and a decline in health.

RIGHT *Milk is nutritious but it is a common allergen.*

Moreover, nutrient-deficient diets typically include large and frequent amounts of common allergens (wheat, milk, yeast, eggs, citrus, alcohol, etc.), and these can impair digestion, irritate the gut lining, and lead to a whole range of food intolerances and allergies.

ABOVE *Wheat, a common allergen, can cause serious digestive problems.*

RIGHT *Imbalanced diets often include too many eggs.*

TODAY'S FOOD CHOICES CREATE TOMORROW'S HEALTH

Extremely bad diets and poor eating habits bring about serious clinical symptoms quickly. A "marginal" diet, however, tends to encourage subclinical deficiencies which do not really materialize as a diagnosed problem for years. Early work

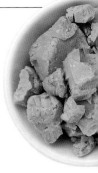

in nutrition demonstrated that nutrient deficiencies caused specific problems, such as lack of vitamin C causing scurvy. However, most nutrients do not have their own specific deficiency symptom, but instead manifest themselves in a variety of seemingly unrelated diseases. Cumulative poor nutrition can create diseases that are not recognized as nutritionally-related disorders, but this is exactly what they are. Subtle health problems become disasters if allowed to continue for years. The phrase "we are what we eat" should really be "we are what we ate a while ago."

ABOVE *Yeast contains vital vitamins and minerals, but it can trigger allergies.*

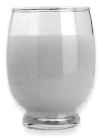

ABOVE *Vitamin C must be taken daily, but citrus fruit can be an irritant.*

The biochemical beginnings of ill health

THE DETERIORATION IN *health leading to many different ailments often has a common starting point. The beginnings of poor health appear to be linked to a breakdown in the way essential nutrients work, which then leads to biochemical imbalance in the body.*

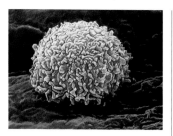

ABOVE *The efficiency of body cells, like this white blood cell, depends on nutrient intake.*

Despite the chemical similarity of some essential nutrients (sodium and potassium, or calcium and magnesium), their biochemical activity is very different – they have quite separate functions. If there is a breakdown in this basic "separation" principle, then a biochemical imbalance occurs which leads to poor health.

Furthermore, if essential nutrient intake falls below the optimum level, the ability of body cells to retain important nutrients and expel other substances starts to fail, and the tissues become more acidic (toxic) than they should be. At the same time, those areas of the body which need to be acidic, such as the stomach (for proper digestion of proteins), become less so. In such cases, protein is not digested fully, and then amino acids (protein end-products) are not adequately absorbed. In addition, the lining of the intestines becomes irritated by the undigested food passing through. Unhelpful bacteria are encouraged to proliferate, leading to "dysbiosis," often manifested as bloating of the lower abdomen, discomfort and/or pain, and excessive "wind." Irritation of the intestinal lining can create a condition known as "leaky gut," where the weakened lining allows partially digested materials to enter the blood-stream directly and initiate an immune response. This may lead to food intolerance or allergy.

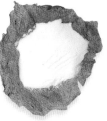

ABOVE *Calcium is an essential mineral for human life.*

LEFT *Broccoli is a good source of calcium.*

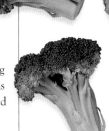

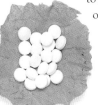

LEFT *Magnesium supplementation is often necessary, especially in the elderly.*

THE STOMACH

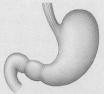

ABOVE *The stomach needs to be an acidic environment for the digestion of proteins.*

COMMON FACTORS IN DISEASE DEVELOPMENT

Most diseases, conditions, and ailments (barring accidents and trauma), are brought about by one, or a combination, of four main factors stemming from biochemical imbalance:

• poor digestion (from incorrect levels of stomach acid and/or poor digestive enzyme production)

• food intolerance and allergy (by frequent consumption of irritating foods)

• nutrient deficiency (from low intake of nutrients and/or poor absorption)

• toxic overload (from the inability of the body to eliminate and excrete various poisonous substances).

Restoring the body to health

THE OVERALL EFFECT of biochemical imbalance is lower body energy, an inefficient metabolism, and the start of malfunctioning. These common conditions may then develop further into specific diseases, not all of which appear to be related directly to faults in the digestion and absorption of food. To restore the body to health, nutritional healing begins by looking at the common factors in disease development (see page 11).

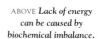

ABOVE *Lack of energy can be caused by biochemical imbalance.*

Healing is brought about by introducing gradually a range of dietary improvements in five main ways:

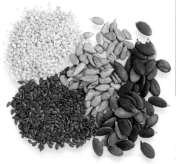

LEFT *Seeds formed an important part of the diet of early humans.*

• Correcting faulty digestion and eliminating food intolerances by the combining of appropriate foods, and by observation of reactions to different food groups.
• Decreasing toxic overload by increasing the amount of nutritious food, and reducing the amount of rich and over-processed foods.

• Releasing healing energy for elimination of toxins by choosing foods from our "primitive" diet (see page 14).

• Encouraging intestinal conditions which will improve absorption of important minerals, vitamins, amino acids, essential fatty acids, and other essential components, by rebalancing the intestinal bacteria.

• Identifying and supporting weakened, overburdened, or exhausted organs by correct use of nutritional supplements. Lifestyle changes may also be needed; for example, increasing the amount of exercise.

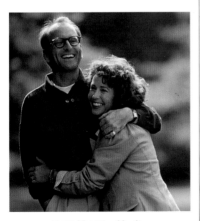

ABOVE **Nutritional healing leads to a more fulfilling quality of life.**

RATE OF IMPROVEMENT

Gradual change rather than drastic measures leads to a more permanent improvement in health. This approach means, of course, that the benefits of nutritional healing may not occur as quickly as by more conventional medical treatment, and patience is required. Nevertheless, on a general basis, you should begin to reap the benefits within two to four weeks from the start of your healing program. The rate of improvement depends on the length of time you have had your symptoms, how committed you are to your new program, the types and quality of supplements you use, and the improvements in other lifestyle areas.

It takes time to optimize digestive function, remove toxins, and nourish the body properly; a health problem that has been decades in the making, is unlikely to be resolved instantly. However, perseverance with a new food program – based on our primitive diet – will reward you a hundredfold.

Our primitive diet

THE EARLIEST HUMANS *were thought to be primarily meat eaters, with seeds, nuts, fruit, and roots making up the remainder of the diet. Fish and other seafood was probably introduced around 25,000 years ago, and 20,000 years after that the early hunter-gatherer humans started to utilize grains.*

LEFT **Meat has formed part of the human diet since the earliest times.**

The wild game that was consumed would have been low in fat (around five percent, as opposed to present day farmed meat of around 30 percent), and probably contained around five times the level of polyunsaturated fats. This primitive diet is likely to have had a polyunsaturated fat content of around three times that of saturated fat. The situation is reversed in our present time. Estimates also indicate that potassium was consumed in amounts ten to fifteen times greater than

ABOVE **Fruit has always been a mainstay of human well-being.**

ABOVE **Humans have eaten seafood for 25,000 years.**

sodium (whereas now we consume around five times more sodium than potassium), and that only one-third of the amount of fiber and one-tenth of the vitamin C eaten by primitive humans is eaten by modern man. To give any animal a diet very different from that which was employed during a major part of its evolution and expect it to remain healthy is extremely foolish. Diseases are bound to occur, and this is exactly what is happening in the developed world.

BELOW **Nuts provide essential minerals.**

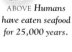

CULTURAL DIETS

For every human culture there is a specific way of selecting, preparing, cooking, and eating food. Some of these "cultural diets" have been around for centuries, others are more recent. Because of different body chemistries, it takes time for people to become accustomed to new dietary practices, but the longer a group remains on its cultural diet, the more each individual within the group will become acclimatized to it. Conversely, dramatic changes are likely to produce rapid development of degenerative diseases. We see evidence of this in people from other parts of the world who take on a Western diet and, along with it, degenerative disease.

ITALIAN

Olives and olive oil form an important part of the Italian diet, as do pasta and cured meats. The Italians like to use fresh herbs, especially basil.

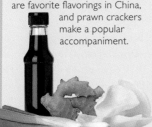

INDIAN

Indian food is noted for its use of spices. Chilies add the heat, and many of the dishes are vegetarian. Rice and a variety of breads are staples.

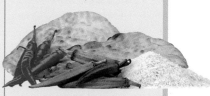

CHINESE

Soy sauce, ginger, and scallions are favorite flavorings in China, and prawn crackers make a popular accompaniment.

FRENCH

French cuisine is world-famous. The best use is made of fresh ingredients, usually served with a glass of wine.

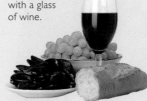

Modern Western diet

IT IS LIKELY *that an appreciation of primitive nutrition, cultural habits, and the variations in individual biochemistry are the basis for the involvement of sound nutrition in the healing of many of the chronic diseases of our time, such as heart disease, diabetes, arthritis, cancer, and many others.*

Besides these considerations, several other factors in modern nutrition are likely to play a part in our escalating ill-health. They are: food processing, convenience foods, pollution, and excessive calorie intake.

FOOD PROCESSING

The processing of foods, such as the refining of flour to increase shelf-life, began at the end of the 19th century.

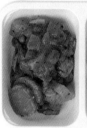 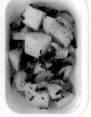

BELOW LEFT **Essential nutrients are reduced by food processing.**

ABOVE **Convenience foods contain added chemical substances.**

CONVENIENCE FOODS

These "new" foods have come into being as a further development in the technology of producing food that is easy to distribute, store, and prepare in the home. To make these "foods" longer-lasting, more colorful, and appealing (since many natural

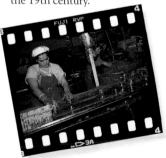

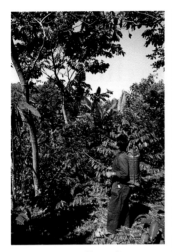

ABOVE *Chemical pesticides find their way into our food and bodies.*

POLLUTION

Because of an increased need for the supply of "raw materials" in order to meet food demand, modern agricultural practices include the use of massive amounts of chemical fertilizers and pesticides.

Some of these chemicals, and their breakdown products, find their way into our food, and ultimately into our bodies.

Many of these substances interfere drastically with our metabolism.

colors and flavors have been processed out), chemical substances are added. Some of these can be harmful to certain susceptible individuals.

Moreover, although we are assured that each food additive has undergone rigorous tests to ensure its safety, most present-day food additives have not been tested together (as they would appear in food). As their synergistic effects – the effect of them in combination – are therefore mostly unknown, they are best avoided.

EXCESSIVE CALORIE INTAKE

People in the West are said to be "overfed and undernourished." Although our total food intake can be excessive, the quality of food is often so poor that the supply of essential nutrients is totally inadequate. Despite soaring and unprecedented levels of obesity in many developed countries (a serious cause for concern), we are actually suffering from malnutrition. In contrast, some developing countries with insufficient food supplies to sustain health suffer from true under-nutrition.

Imbalances in the Western diet

COMPARED TO ONLY *two or three hundred years ago, today's "Western" food contains many substances which our body chemistry is unable to metabolize, especially when intake of vitamins and minerals is so poor. Excessive consumption of refined carbohydrates, sugar, salt, saturated fat (fatty meats and dairy food), and highly-processed fats (hydrogenated and trans fatty acids), destabilizes the system even more.*

It is easy to see why the Western diet is believed to be a major cause of cancer, heart disease, and osteoporosis. It is now accepted that a deficient or excessive diet is a major risk factor in heart disease and cancer – two of our modern primary killers – but how many more diseases might be attributed to chemicals and pollutants in our food?

Also, recent information suggests that a lack of less well-known nutrients, e.g., essential fatty acids, may cause illness,

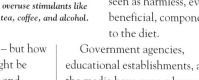

ABOVE **Western diets overuse stimulants like tea, coffee, and alcohol.**

especially when poorly balanced with too much saturated fat. In addition, Western diets tend to overuse stimulants such as tea, coffee, and alcohol, yet these are seen as harmless, even beneficial, components to the diet.

Government agencies, educational establishments, and the media have gone a long way to get the message across to eat a low salt, low fat, high fiber diet. But the imbalance caused by over-processed, polluted, and nutrient-deficient food,

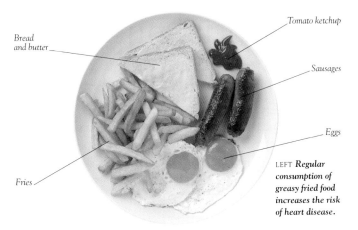

Bread and butter

Tomato ketchup

Sausages

Eggs

Fries

LEFT *Regular consumption of greasy fried food increases the risk of heart disease.*

combined with what appears to be a general malaise of deficient digestion and poor absorption, is yet to be proclaimed. Only when more accurate information is freely available will a greater number of people be better able to make more wholesome choices. By using sound nutrition and a healthier lifestyle, many Western diseases would be preventable and, perhaps, even curable.

DRAWBACKS OF THE WESTERN DIET

- too much saturated and/or processed fat, but insufficient essential fatty acids
- too much salt, but an insufficient range and amount of essential minerals
- too much sugar and white flour, but insufficient fiber
- too many processed foods with their consequent essential nutrient loss
- too many stimulants (tea, coffee, alcohol)
- potentially harmful insecticides, pesticides, herbicides, and additives

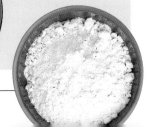

RIGHT *Bran contains the fiber and essential nutrients lacking in white flour.*

Essential nutrient requirements

OUR NUTRITIONAL REQUIREMENTS *vary according to the demands being made on our digestion and metabolism by the food we eat, and our general health, age, and lifestyle – all things that have a significant effect on our individual biochemistry.*

In addition, anyone with an inherited metabolic defect, or who exercises excessively, or is pregnant will have nutrient requirements far above the "normal." There is an optimum range of nutrient intake for each one of us, but because the range of nutrients is so wide and our biochemical differences so great, it is almost impossible to have a clearly defined amount calculated for each of the 50 or so nutrients we know of.

ABOVE *Busy lifestyles make demands on our nutrient intake.*

FACTORS AFFECTING NUTRITIONAL STATUS

• The quality of the food you eat; high quality organic food is always the best choice even if it costs a little more.
• The quantity of food you eat; smaller quantities of nutrient-dense food are much better than consuming large quantities of processed food.
• Digestive and absorptive capability; good digestion and absorption will allow greater uptake of essential nutrients, providing the most benefit.

RIGHT *Active and growing children have different nutritional needs from the elderly.*

FACTORS RELATING TO BIOCHEMICAL INDIVIDUALITY

- **AGE:** the older we get, the more essential nutrients we require, but fewer calories.
- **STAGE OF GROWTH:** the faster we are growing, the more essential nutrients we require (obviously only applies to children).
- **GENDER:** men and women (especially if pregnant or breastfeeding) of similar age can have different requirements of the same nutrients.
- **STATE OF GENERAL HEALTH:** essential nutrients are more easily lost, and harder to replenish when we are ill, especially if appetite is poor.
- **STRESS LEVELS:** stressful situations can deplete the body of essential nutrients very quickly.
- **ACTIVITY LEVEL:** the more active you are, the greater the nutrient demand.
- **STIMULANT INTAKE:** the more tea, coffee, alcohol, etc. in the diet, the greater the nutrient demand.
- **TOXIC LEVELS:** the taking of any drugs, smoking, or working/living in a polluted environment will increase nutrient demand.

FIRST STEPS IN DIETARY IMPROVEMENT

- Eat nutrient-dense foods (unprocessed, wholefoods); avoid processed and refined food, and food additives.
- Eat organic food, and drink filtered or bottled water.
- Cut down on stimulants (tea, coffee).
- Avoid saturated animal fat, but eat foods containing essential fatty acids (e.g., pumpkin and sunflower seeds).

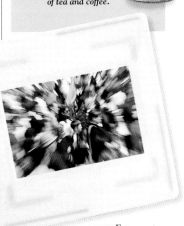

RIGHT *Drink filtered or bottled water instead of tea and coffee.*

ABOVE *Extreme stress can quickly lead to nutrient deficiency.*

Acid/alkaline balance

ONE FURTHER IMPORTANT ASPECT *of nutrition is the acid/alkaline balance in the body. Under normal conditions, signs of over-acidity (poor mental function, fatigue, arthritic disorders, muscle aches and pains) should not occur because the body is able to "buffer" any excess acid via alkaline reserves in blood and bone. Modern living, however, with its excessive concentrated protein (e.g., meat) intake and high stress levels, can exhaust this buffering capacity.*

When this happens, excess acidity has to be neutralized by a "bicarbonate buffer system," which requires sodium and calcium. When blood reserves are used up, the body calls on calcium from the bones. Thus there is a link between excessive protein consumption and bone density loss. This acid-buffering system needs a supply of alkaline minerals from our food, and so our diet needs to be made up of around 80 percent alkali-forming and neutral foods, and only 20 percent acid-forming foods.

The natural acidity of food and its ability to become "acid-forming" when metabolized in the body are two different things. When food is metabolized a mineral ash remains. When this ash is rich in calcium, sodium, potassium, and magnesium it is "alkali-forming" but when it contains large amounts of chlorine, sulfur, and phosphorus, it is "acid-forming."

ABOVE *To determine pH levels, pH paper strips are used.*

BELOW *A pH below seven indicates an acid; above seven is alkaline.*

| 8.1 | 7.8 | 7.5 | 7.2 | 6.9 | 6.6 | 6.3 | 6.0 |

ALKALINE

Alkaline ash-forming foods
All fruits *(except cranberries, plums, and prunes)*, milk, egg white, molasses, some nuts *(almonds and brazils)*, all vegetables *(including green beans, peas, and potatoes)*, sea vegetables *(seaweed)*, fungi *(mushrooms)*, sprouted seeds and some pulses (legumes) *(kidney beans, azuki beans, soybeans)*, tofu, millet, tamari, miso and salt, coffee.

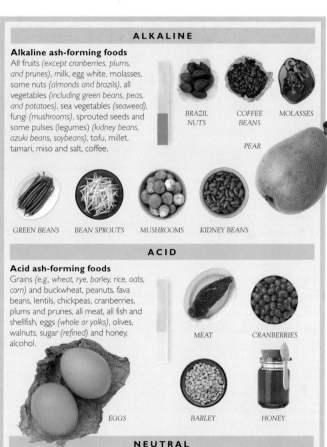

BRAZIL NUTS

COFFEE BEANS

MOLASSES

PEAR

GREEN BEANS

BEAN SPROUTS

MUSHROOMS

KIDNEY BEANS

ACID

Acid ash-forming foods
Grains *(e.g., wheat, rye, barley, rice, oats, corn)* and buckwheat, peanuts, fava beans, lentils, chickpeas, cranberries, plums and prunes, all meat, all fish and shellfish, eggs *(whole or yolks)*, olives, walnuts, sugar *(refined)* and honey, alcohol.

MEAT

CRANBERRIES

EGGS

BARLEY

HONEY

NEUTRAL

Neutral foods
Yogurt, seeds *(sesame, pumpkin, and sunflower)*, butter, margarine, some cheeses, tea.

PUMPKIN SEEDS

BUTTER

YOGURT

CHEESE

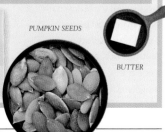

What is a well-balanced diet?

A WELL-BALANCED *diet is one which supplies the body with all the nutrients it requires, in the correct proportions for optimum health. The New Pyramid program is the foundation for healthy eating: it gives you a sound basis upon which to build your own unique program, providing for as many as possible of your biochemical requirements.*

The New Pyramid program requires some refinement of the conventional "balanced diet," which takes no account of the types and variety of foods within each food group necessary for a healthy balance; possible nutrient depletion in processed foods; or the genetic differences, changing needs, or state of health of the individual. All of these factors require attention if we are to eat optimally.

Also, because of modern food production techniques, even fresh fruit and vegetables do not contain the levels of nutrients they did in the past. Analysis of some nutrient levels has indicated, on average, a decline of around 22 percent in mineral content of fruit and vegetables over the last 50 years. It has even been found that some supermarket oranges contain no vitamin C whatsoever. It is quite possible that the average person consuming a conventional "balanced diet" is deficient in several essential nutrients.

This means the "balanced diet" needs to be re-examined to give more precise information on the relative amounts of each type of food within each of the main food groups – carbohydrates, proteins, and fats. The New Pyramid program visually displays the ratio of all the important foods and their acid/alkaline tendencies in a triangular diagram.

THE NEW FOOD PYRAMID

The New Pyramid program balances carbohydrate with protein, and attempts to restore acid/alkaline balance. It is designed to contain a good mix of nutrient-dense foods.

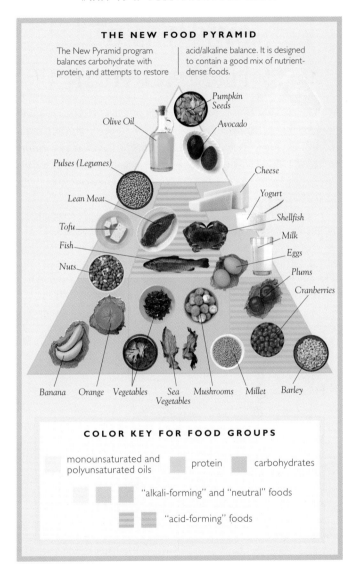

Pumpkin Seeds

Olive Oil

Avocado

Pulses (Legumes)

Cheese

Lean Meat

Yogurt

Tofu

Shellfish

Fish

Milk

Nuts

Eggs

Plums

Cranberries

Banana   Orange   Vegetables   Sea Vegetables   Mushrooms   Millet   Barley

COLOR KEY FOR FOOD GROUPS

monounsaturated and polyunsaturated oils   protein   carbohydrates

"alkali-forming" and "neutral" foods

"acid-forming" foods

New Pyramid carbohydrates

AT THE BASE *of the pyramid, making up the largest portion of your food at around 40 percent of calorie intake, are the fruits, vegetables, and wholegrain carbohydrates. Carbohydrates are needed by the body mainly as an energy source, and to supply fiber for intestinal health and proper elimination of wastes.*

Vegetables, fruit, unrefined whole grains (wheat, rye, corn, oats, barley, rice, millet, quinoa), and buckwheat (related to rhubarb), satisfy both these criteria. However, many people find wheat a problem since allergies to it are common, and wheatbran is especially harsh on the intestinal lining. Soluble fibers – cellulose, hemicellulose, and pectins – found in vegetables, fruits, and some grains (such as oats and rice) are therefore a better choice. In addition, fibrous carbohydrates help bulk up the food and keep hunger at bay. This can be particularly useful if you are trying to lose weight.

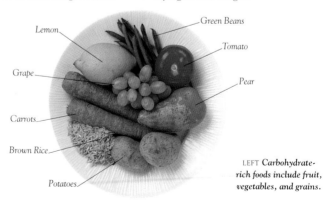

Lemon

Green Beans

Tomato

Grape

Pear

Carrots

Brown Rice

Potatoes

LEFT **Carbohydrate-rich foods include fruit, vegetables, and grains.**

SUGARS AND STARCHES

Energy-giving carbohydrates comprise the sugars glucose and fructose (fruit sugar), maltose (malt), sucrose ("sugar") and lactose (milk sugar), and the starches found in potatoes, parsnips, and in grains and their products (breakfast cereals, pasta, bread). Bear in mind that refined carbohydrates (white bread, "sugar," sugar-rich cakes and cookies, and pastries) have no place here, and to make sure that you have a good mixture of the important minerals and vitamins within the "complex" (unrefined) carbohydrates, you should select a variety and not stick to only one or two.

HIGH GLYCEMIC FOODS

Some grains and their products (bread, pasta, processed breakfast cereals), and some starchy vegetables are "high glycaemic foods." This means they cause fast release of sugar into the bloodstream and can upset the insulin release mechanism. These foods need to be kept at a low level in any diet to prevent blood sugar imbalances. Because of this, the daily servings of "high-glycemic" foods are kept low in the New Pyramid diet. Having only minimal amounts of wholegrain carbohydrate will also keep acid-forming foods in balance. However, whole grains contain many essential vitamins and minerals, so it is important that they are not cut from the diet altogether.

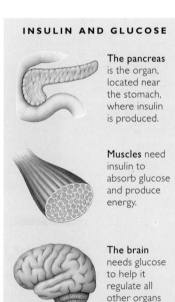

INSULIN AND GLUCOSE

The pancreas is the organ, located near the stomach, where insulin is produced.

Muscles need insulin to absorb glucose and produce energy.

The brain needs glucose to help it regulate all other organs and systems.

New Pyramid proteins

THE NEXT LEVEL *upward contains the proteins, which should make up a maximum of 30 percent of your calorie intake. Proteins are needed for growth, repair, and replacement of tissues. They are made up of around 20 or so different "amino acids." Eight of these are essential because the body cannot make them from other amino acids, and three are conditionally essential (i.e., they can become essential if diet is poor).*

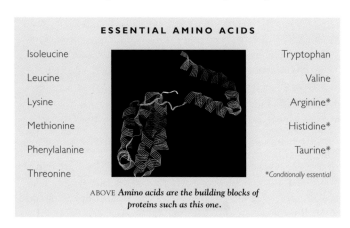

ESSENTIAL AMINO ACIDS

Isoleucine	Tryptophan
Leucine	Valine
Lysine	Arginine*
Methionine	Histidine*
Phenylalanine	Taurine*
Threonine	*Conditionally essential

ABOVE **Amino acids are the building blocks of proteins such as this one.**

Proteins also function biochemically, being important for enzymes (biological catalysts), some hormones and their associates the "prostaglandins" (chemical messengers), antibodies to fight disease, neurotransmitters (chemicals needed for the transmission of nervous impulses), and other specific structural roles.

PROTEIN SOURCES

We obviously need good quality protein in our diet but excessive intake of animal protein, in particular, can cause acidosis of the tissues, and overworking of the liver and kidneys. In addition, if animal protein is not organic, you are likely to be consuming fair amounts of antibiotics, hormone residues, and other pollutants. Also since protein excess to bodily requirements cannot be stored, it is converted to fat. So too much dietary protein will lead to overweight.

As a general rule, dairy foods (even from an organic source) are problematical for two reasons. Firstly, like wheat, milk (particularly cow's milk) can cause allergy in susceptible people; secondly, milk contains saturated fat. For both these reasons, dairy foods should feature minimally in any healthy diet. A large proportion of fatty meat and red meat, although containing good quality protein, should also be restricted because of the saturated fat levels. Fish is a better choice of protein for flesh-eaters, and tofu is an excellent protein for vegetarians and vegans.

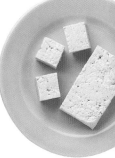

ABOVE *Tofu is a healthy source of protein, not only for vegetarians.*

Select a wide range from (in descending order of importance), oily fish, lean meat, tofu, lentils, beans, seeds, nuts, dairy food, and eggs. Always balance animal and plant protein if you are a meat eater, and for two or three days a week take your protein quota from the pulses (legumes), seeds, nuts, and tofu.

If you are a fish and dairy consuming vegetarian, then just leave out the meat; if you are a strict vegetarian or a vegan, you can attain balance by having equal amounts of tofu and pulses (legumes) with smaller amounts of grains, nuts, and seeds.

LEFT *An adequate supply of protein is essential for a healthy body.*

New Pyramid fats and oils

THE TOP OF *the food pyramid contains the fats and oils. These account for around 30 percent of calorie intake, but as they contain more than twice the number of calories of either protein or carbohydrate, you only need very small servings to obtain your fat quota. For example, if you are having a meal containing 3oz (75g) of fish (or tofu) plus a large salad, you would fulfill your fat quota from half a teaspoon of olive oil, or a few seeds.*

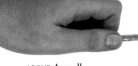

ABOVE **A small quantity of olive oil will provide your fat quota.**

Fats are made up of a combination of fatty acids. There are two major groups of essential polyunsaturated fatty acids: omega 3 (linolenic acid), found in pumpkin seeds and flax seeds (edible linseeds), and omega 6 (linoleic acid), found in sunflower and sesame seeds. Many processed foods, particularly polyunsaturated margarine, supply omega 6 with none, or very little, omega 3.

This imbalance may be involved in the continued rise in cardiovascular disease, despite the popular change to polyunsaturated margarines.

Vital body processes depend on a good supply and correct balance of these essential fatty acids, so much so that typical Western diseases such as heart disease, stroke, obesity, and cancer are possibly caused as much by lack of essential fatty acids as by diets high in saturated fat. Processed dairy products can contain two further substances – hydrogenated fats and trans fatty acids – and these also appear to be implicated in disease, since the body is unable to metabolize them. Butter or a good quality margarine can be used, but sparingly.

Fish oils and mono-unsaturated oils are included in this pyramid level. Fish oils (from your fish intake) supply EHA and DHA – two more important fatty acids. The best monounsaturated oil is olive oil, now well known through studies of Mediterranean diets for its apparent health-giving properties, particularly for prevention of heart disease.

NEW PYRAMID TREATS

No one is going to stick to a diet that doesn't allow any treats. The odd cake, chocolate, or glass of wine is going to do you no harm, but bear in mind that the health-giving foods within this program should be your major choices. When you do decide to have a treat, count it as part of your carbohydrate quota.

HEART

The heart is the hardest working organ in the human body. We rely on it to work efficiently every moment of every day and any disorder that stops it pumping properly can be a threat to life. Diet is recognized as being a major factor in maintaining a healthy heart and preventing disease of the coronary arteries.

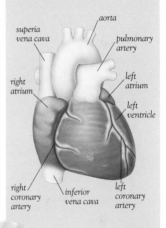

aorta

superia vena cava

pulmonary artery

right atrium

left atrium

left ventricle

right coronary artery

inferior vena cava

left coronary artery

ABOVE **A healthy heart can be relied on to pump blood at a steady rate with no conscious assistance.**

LEFT *Occasional treats can be part of your carbohydrate quota.*

The New Pyramid program

THE TABLES BELOW *will help you construct your well-balanced eating plan. The first gives information on serving sizes (to keep carbohydrates, proteins, and fats in balance); the second shows how many portions of each food group you need each day; the third indicates the ratios of foods (from within the subdivisions of the three food groups), using the codes from the first table.*

THE NEW PYRAMID SERVING SIZES			
FOOD GROUP	**FOOD**	**CODE**	**SERVING SIZE**
Carbohydrate	Vegetables (*except potatoes*)	C1	4oz (100g)
	Sprouted seeds; mushrooms	C1	4oz (100g)
	Fruit	C1	2oz (50g)
	Whole grains, breads, pasta, and starchy vegetables, e.g., potatoes	C2	1oz (27g)
Protein	Oily fish (*includes 1 fat serving*);	P1	1½oz (40g)
	Shellfish	P1	1½oz (40g)
	Lean meat e.g., chicken	P1	1oz (27g)
	Tofu	P1	3oz (80g)
	Dairy: cottage cheese	P1	2oz (50g)
	hard cheese (*includes 1 fat serving*)	P1	1oz (27g)
	yogurt	P1	3oz (80g)
	milk (skimmed)	P1	3oz (80g)
	Eggs (*includes 2 fat servings*)	P1	1oz (27g)
	Nuts (*includes 2 fat servings*)	P2	1½oz (40g)
	Seeds (*includes 1 fat serving*)	P2	2oz (50g)
	Pulses (*includes 1 carbohydrate serving*)	P2	2oz (50g)
Fat	Olive oil; sesame oil; Sunflower oil; butter	F1	½tsp (2.5ml)
	Nuts (*includes some protein*)	F2	1tsp (5ml)
	Seeds (*includes some protein*)	F2	1½ tsp (7.5ml)
	Peanut butter, tahini, nut butters (*includes some protein*)	F3	1tsp (5ml)
	Avocado	F3	1oz (27g)
	Fish oils (*included in protein list*)		

THE NEW PYRAMID DAILY SERVINGS
(related to body size and levels of activity)

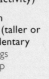

Small to average
size, sedentary
Five servings
of each group

Greater than
average size (taller or
heavier), sedentary
Seven servings
of each group

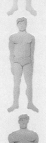

Small to average size,
moderately active
Seven servings
of each group

Greater than average
size, moderately active
Nine servings
of each group

Small to average
size, very active
Nine servings
of each group

Greater than average
size, very active
Eleven servings
of each group

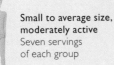

NUMBER OF DAILY SERVINGS	CARBOHYDRATES		PROTEIN		OILS		
	C1	C2	P1	P2	F1	F2	F3
5	4	1	2	3	2	2	1
7	5	2	3	4	2	3	2
9	5	4*	5**	4	3	3	3
11	6	5*	6**	5	4	4	3

RATIO OF DAILY SERVINGS

*As serving size increases, use more millet and potato to keep acidity low
**As serving size increases, use more tofu and/or fish to keep dairy foods low

Vitamins

VITAMINS AND MINERALS *are called "micronutrients" since, despite their essential nature, they are only required in very small amounts, unlike fats, protein, and carbohydrates – the "macronutrients" – which are needed in fairly large amounts.*

Vitamins are not structural components of the body, unlike some minerals (e.g., calcium in the bones), but have a biochemical function. In conjunction with enzymes, they allow chemical reactions within the cell to proceed. They are involved in energy metabolism, hormonal balance, immune function, the skin and connective tissue, blood vessel protection, brain function and the transmission of nervous impulses, and many other bodily functions.

The table below gives some idea of the variability of their actions, and the best sources.

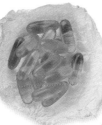

ABOVE *Cod liver oil is an excellent source of vitamin A.*

VITAMIN SOURCES AND FUNCTIONS

VITAMIN	FUNCTION IN BODY	BEST SOURCES
A (retinol)	Retina of the eye; mucous membranes	Liver, fish liver oils (Do not eat when pregnant)
A (B-carotene)	As above; antioxidant	Carrots, dark-green vegetables
B1 (thiamine)	Metabolism of carbohydrates; nervous system	Whole grains, seeds, beans, nuts, fish
B2 (riboflavin)	Metabolism of fats, proteins, and carbohydrates; toxin removal	Lean meat, fish, wheatgerm, broccoli and other greens, pulses

VITAMIN SOURCES AND FUNCTIONS

VITAMIN	FUNCTION IN BODY	BEST SOURCES
B3 *(niacin)*	As B2; red blood cells; some hormones,	Liver, fish, poultry, peanuts, whole grains, eggs
B5 *(pantothenate)*	Neurotransmitter; glycogen and fatty acid production	As above
B6 **(Pyridoxal-5-phosphate)**	Protein metabolism; hemoglobin production; antibodies	Wheatgerm, seeds, poultry, lamb, fish, avocados, oats, soybeans, walnuts, bananas, cabbage
B12 *(cyanocobalamin)*	Cellular functioning; nervous system	Liver, oysters, poultry, fish, eggs, fermented foods (e.g., miso)
Folate	Protein metabolism; cell division; nervous system; neural tube development	Wheatgerm, dark-green leafy vegetables, beans, egg yolks, nuts, wholewheat, salmon
Biotin	Glycogen and fatty acid metabolism; prostaglandins; skin, hair, and nerves	Liver, sardines, egg yolks, soy, whole grains, nuts, and beans
C *(ascorbic acid)*	Collagen formation; skin; immune function	Guava, Brussels sprouts, blackcurrants, cranberries, kiwi fruit, bell peppers, peas, broccoli, tomatoes, citrus fruits
D *(cholecalci-ferol)*	Calcium and phosphorus absorption; bone growth	Fish liver oils, sunlight on skin
E *(tocopherol)*	Antioxidant; anticoagulant	Wheatgerm oil, wheatgerm, soybean oil, olive oil, egg yolk, liver, nuts, seeds
K *(phylloquinone)*	Blood-clotting mechanism	Raw cauliflower, green leafy vegetables, good bacteria in intestines
Choline and Inositol	Neurotransmitters; nervous system; calcium metabolism; insulin activity	Soy lecithin, egg yolks, liver, fish, whole grains, nuts

Minerals

MINERALS, LIKE VITAMINS, *are essential for just about every process within the body. However, unlike vitamins, some minerals become incorporated into body structures, e.g., calcium, magnesium, and phosphorus in bones. Others are similar to vitamins in that they help metabolism, acting as coenzymes; e.g., magnesium, zinc, iron, and copper.*

ABOVE **Figs provide the body with potassium.**

The essential minerals in food make up only around four percent of body tissues. Calcium, magnesium, phosphorus, sodium, chloride, and potassium – collectively called the "macrominerals" – make up a major portion of this amount. They are largely involved with the structural part of the skeleton and the teeth, and as electrolytes, balancing negative and positive charges in the blood and tissue fluids. Yet others have very specific functions, such as the role of iron as the central element in each molecule of hemoglobin.

As with vitamins, correct nutrition is vital to obtain sufficient amounts of these within the body because they are not as abundant as

ABOVE **Another macromineral, calcium, is found in yogurt.**

the "macronutrients." The twelve or so "trace minerals" are only needed in very tiny amounts. It is even more crucial to ensure that this latter group of nutrients is adequately supplied by the diet.

Many minerals are co-workers, so that the absence of one mineral severely disrupts the functions of others, and ultimately the workings of the metabolism.

The table opposite demonstrates their comprehensive list of functions, together with suggested food sources.

THE MACROMINERALS

MINERAL	FUNCTION IN BODY	BEST SOURCES
Calcium	Bones; teeth; nerves; cells	Canned fish (bones), whitebait, nuts, yogurt, milk, sesame seeds, broccoli, tofu, cheese
Magnesium	Bones; teeth; cofactor for many enzymes; muscles; nerves	Millet, lima beans, black-eyed beans, soybeans, seeds, wheatgerm, fish, nuts, dark-green vegetables, buckwheat, brown rice
Phosphorus	Bones; teeth; red cells	Meats, fish, wholegrains, nuts
Potassium	Heart rate; water balance; nerves	Tomato paste, dried apricots, figs, bananas, pumpkin seeds, almonds, soybeans, potatoes, green-leafy vegetables, fish, avocados, beans
Sodium	Electrolyte; nerves	Plentiful, even in low-salt diet
Chloride	As above; stomach acid	As above

TRACE MINERALS

MINERAL	FUNCTION IN BODY	BEST SOURCES
Boron	Bones; hormones	Alfalfa, cabbage, lettuce, peas, soybeans, almonds, hazelnuts, apples, prunes
Chromium	Glucose metabolism; fatty acid and protein metabolism	Wholegrains, shellfish, liver, seeds, nuts, black pepper, molasses
Cobalt	Vitamin B12 structure	Liver, kidney, oysters, meat, fish, sea vegetables, miso
Copper	Enzymes; blood; hormones	Offal, seafood, cherries, cocoa, cashew nuts, olives
Fluorine	Bones; teeth	Fish, seafood, black tea
Iodine	Thyroxine hormone	Haddock, mackerel, cod, live yogurt, seaweed, iodized salt
Iron	Hemoglobin	Cockles, molasses, cocoa, liver, meat, wheatgerm, prunes, nuts, seaweed
Manganese	Bones; cartilage; glucose metabolism; antioxidant production; brain; nerves	Whole grains, rice bran, wheatgerm, nuts, black tea, ginger, cloves, green vegetables
Molybdenum	Enzyme systems; antioxidant; iron utilization; reproduction	Whole grains, legumes, liver, buckwheat, wheatgerm, sunflower seeds, beans
Selenium	Antioxidant; thyroid action	Nuts, cashews, molasses, soybeans, tuna, seafood, meat, whole grains, wheatgerm
Silicon	Bones; skin; hair; membranes	Seaweed, whole grains
Zinc	Reproductive system; enzymes; stomach acid; wound healing	Oysters, seafood, popcorn, eggs, sesame and pumpkin seeds, fish, wheatgerm, meat

Nickel, Vanadium, Tin, and Germanium are also needed by the body, but their exact roles are still being researched.

Proper use of supplements

THERE ARE MANY *nutritional supplements on the market nowadays, making it very difficult to choose the right ones. In general, it is best to self-prescribe only the multiformulas (multiminerals and multivitamins) which cover a broad spectrum of nutrients in one capsule or tablet, since taking isolated nutrient supplements can have a disastrous effect on the metabolism's fine tuning, and may be toxic in large doses.*

ABOVE *Seek advice if you're not sure which supplements to take.*

Even if you buy multiformula supplements from a health food shop, you may still find that there is an endless variety to choose from: some excellent, high quality products, others that are very near useless. Generally, you get what you pay for. Some prices may seem excessive, but usually this reflects the high level of research, preparation, and quality control that goes into their production.

If you feel that your health problems require specific supplementation, it would be safer (and cheaper in the long run) to obtain the help of a nutritional therapist. To get the very best from supplements, follow the few basic principles given here to maximize uptake.

LEFT *Take supplements with water and avoid drinking tea or coffee for 30 minutes.*

IMPROVING THE ABSORPTION OF SUPPLEMENTS

• Keep alcohol and supplements separate – alcohol will leach nutrients immediately.

• Avoid drinking tea and coffee at mealtimes, or when taking your supplement – these drinks also have a leaching effect.

• If you cannot refrain from smoking, do not smoke for at least 30 minutes either side of a meal or taking supplements – the chemicals in tobacco smoke have a leaching effect on nutrients and use up antioxidants in the process.

• Take time out to eat slowly – stressful activities (like eating too fast) can shut down digestion, and prevent absorption.

• Fat-soluble vitamins are best taken with meals that contain some fat – this will help "escort" them into the body.

• Keep your intestines functioning well by eating adequate levels of a good variety of fiber, and live yogurt .

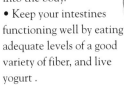

ABOVE *Generally, price gives a fair indication of product quality.*

• Foods high in B vitamins (e.g., cereals), and vitamin B supplements are best taken early in the day, since they "kick-start" the metabolism.

Never take supplements, especially those containing minerals, on an empty stomach (unless advised to do so); they may bring on nausea.

Never take "single" supplements unless under the guidance of a nutritional therapist – metabolism may easily become unbalanced if you do.

Never stop taking supplements suddenly; tail them off gradually so that your body has time to readjust.

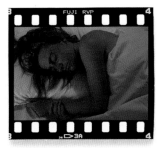

LEFT *Calming supplements like magnesium and zinc are best taken 30 minutes or so before bedtime.*

Antioxidants

ANTIOXIDANTS ARE SUBSTANCES *found in the body, and in food, that protect us from oxidative damage caused by stress, excessive exercise, radiation, pollution, and eating certain processed, fried, or barbecued foods. Oxidation also happens as part of our normal metabolic functioning.*

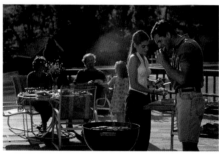

ABOVE *Barbecues are fun occasionally, but too much charred or burnt food can be dangerous.*

Our bodies are equipped with a set of "antioxidant enzymes" to counteract free radical damage. However, if these become overwhelmed, antioxidant nutrients, such as beta-carotene, vitamin E, vitamin C, molybdenum, selenium, zinc, and glutathione, are needed to "mop up" free radicals that escape the antioxidant enzymes in the body.

Oxidative damage is caused by rogue particles called "free radicals." These have been implicated as a central feature in the ageing process; and in diseases such as cardiovascular disease, diabetes, cataracts, high blood pressure, infertility, gum disease, respiratory infections, rheumatoid arthritis, Alzheimer's disease, and even cancer and mental illness.

Antioxidant nutrients are found primarily in fresh fruits and vegetables. Herbs and plant extracts are also included in the list of substances containing excellent ranges of antioxidants. For example, Ginkgo biloba is a particularly efficient scavenger of a free radical called hydroxyl.

EXAMPLES OF ANTIOXIDANTS IN FOOD

- **Anthocyanidins** are found in berries and grapes, particularly in the skins.

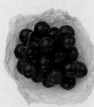

- **Beta-carotenes** are found in orange fruits and vegetables (e.g., apricots and carrots).

- **Lutein,** another powerful carotene antioxidant (it is additionally extremely heat-stable and can survive cooking), is found in many fruits and vegetables, such as spinach and other dark-green vegetables.

- **Bioflavonoids** are found in citrus fruit (particularly the white inner rind), buckwheat, and onions and garlic.

- **Curcumin** is a powerful antioxidant found in mustard, turmeric, yellow peppers, and corn.

- **Proanthocyanidins,** found in green tea and grape seeds, are deemed to be far more potent than vitamin E.

- **Lycopene** is a particularly powerful antioxidant found in tomatoes.

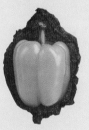

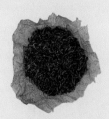

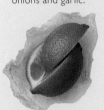

Grapes, apricots, yellow peppers, broccoli, green tea, and limes belong to groups of foods containing different antioxidants.

Phytochemicals

PHYTOCHEMICALS ARE BIOLOGICALLY *active compounds found commonly in everyday wholesome food, such as fruits, vegetables, beans, rice, and even chocolate and red wine! Phytochemicals are closely related to antioxidants and their functions overlap. They are not theoretically classified as nutrients since our lives do not depend on them. Nevertheless, they have been found to play a vital role in our biochemistry and, therefore, have a direct relevance to our health.*

So far, well over a hundred of these substances have been isolated and identified, and many of them appear to have an important regulating effect on hormones and the immune system, and are therefore of great importance in prevention of cancer, improving immune resistance, and in delaying the signs of ageing.

Use the table opposite to help you obtain optimum antioxidant and phytochemical amounts daily.

LEFT *Good health depends upon the complex balance of our body's biochemistry.*

BODY PROTECTORS

This group of substances, important in regulating body systems, is being seen as a major breakthrough in nutritional healing. They are:

Important for cancer protection, forming healthy red blood cells, killing germs, and wound healing.

Useful in preventing the formation of cancer-causing nitrosamines in the gut.

Often rich in phytoestrogens which help with menopausal problems.

ANTIOXIDANT/PHYTOCHEMICAL FOOD CHOICES

These are the best vegetables, fruits, whole grains, seeds, and nuts, to eat as part of your New Pyramid program.

Choose one item from as many groups as possible each week, varying your choice each day.

GROUP 1
Broccoli
Brussels sprouts
Cauliflower

GROUP 2
Spinach
Tomato
Kale

GROUP 3
Sweet potato
Yellow squash
Carrots

GROUP 4
Garlic
Onion
Leeks

GROUP 5
Cabbage
Peas
Sweetcorn

GROUP 6
Radish
Turnip
Horseradish

GROUP 7
Fennel
Alfalfa
Rhubarb

GROUP 8
Cantaloupe
Pawpaw
Mango

GROUP 9
Citrus
Kiwi fruit
Sweet peppers

GROUP 10
Grapes
Berries
Fresh Currants

GROUP 11
Strawberries
Raspberries
Pineapple

GROUP 12
Cress
Sprouted seeds
Sea vegetables

GROUP 13
Mustard
Yellow pepper
Turmeric

GROUP 14
Sunflower seeds
Pumpkin seeds
Mixed nuts

GROUP 15
Black tea
Black pepper
Mixed nuts

GROUP 16
Soybeans
Lentils and beans
Buckwheat

GROUP 17
Olive oil
Wheatgerm
Dried apricots

GROUP 18
Rice bran*
Rice oil*
Barley oil*

* from wholegrain brown rice and barley

43

Beginning the New Pyramid program

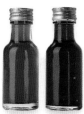

ABOVE **You won't miss the artificial flavorings for long.**

WHEN YOU BEGIN *the New Pyramid program, remember that wholefoods taste different from processed foods – the latter contain many flavorings and flavor-enhancing chemicals. As you begin to consume the foods recommended here, you may find them bland to start with, but after a week or two your taste buds will return to their natural state, and you will be able to savor the natural flavors in these chemical-free wholefoods.*

TEN MAJOR HEALTH CHANGES WITH THE NEW PYRAMID PROGRAM

1 Saturated fat intake will be reduced, and essential fatty acids raised.

2 Protein level will be in line with biochemical demands, and will be obtained from a range of sources.

3 Sugar and salt will be reduced, and natural sugars and mineral salts will be obtained from vegetables and fruits.

4 Intake of all necessary vitamins and minerals will be increased.

5 Intake of important antioxidants and phytochemicals will be increased.

6 Dietary fiber will be obtained from a range of fiber types.

7 Carbohydrate intake will be well balanced and will consist of "complex" types rather than "refined" types.

8 Consumption of convenience foods and artificial additives will be drastically reduced.

9 Intake of environmental toxins and pollutants will be reduced if most of your food is organic.

10 The pH balance will conform more to the 80 percent alkaline/20 percent acid ratio.

GENERAL HINTS FOR
THE NEW PYRAMID PROGRAM

The list below may look somewhat daunting but you'll soon get used to your new food regime and then you'll begin to reap the rewards by feeling and looking much better.

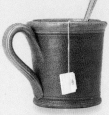

ABOVE **Drink herb and fruit teas or other caffeine-free beverages.**

• Avoid any form of sugar (except fructose), additives, sugar substitutes, refined or processed food.

• Minimize intake of alcohol, coffee, and tea.

• Avoid fried, burnt, or "browned" food, hydrogenated fats and margarines. Use saturated fat very sparingly.

• Eat raw vegetables and sprouted seeds/pulses (legumes) as much as you can.

• Keep dairy foods to a minimum. Instead of cow's milk, try rice, soy, or oat milk, and use soy cream instead of ordinary cream. Live yogurt is the exception; it should be eaten daily for the natural bacteria needed in the intestines.

• Drink 4 to 6 half-pint glasses of water per day, plus diluted fruit juices (1:1 juice to water). Keep citrus juices to a minimum. Have herb tea, fruit tea, rooibosh tea, dandelion coffee, or other coffee substitutes. Consume most of your drinks in between meals to prevent dilution of digestive enzymes.

• Supplement your diet with a high potency, good quality, multivitamin/multimineral and 1,000mg (1g) vitamin C a day.

• Eat when you are hungry and not out of habit.

• Wherever possible, eat organic food.

• Don't eat when you are in a hurry, stressed, or upset.

• Chew food thoroughly.

• Treat all fats and oils with great care. Rancidity (producing free radicals) occurs quickly and can be brought about by air, temperature, light, or contact with metals.

RIGHT **Store butter in glass or china rather than metal.**

Diets for health

THE NEW PYRAMID *program can be used as a basis for the development of other related diet programs designed for healing of specific ailments and problems, and for helping to restore the body to maximum health.*

IMPROVING DIGESTION AND ABSORPTION

This program is designed to improve digestion, soothe the gut lining, provide essential fatty acids, and re-establish helpful gut bacteria. It can be continued for as long as you wish.

• Consume only fresh food.

• Eat plenty of fruit, fibrous vegetables, and brown rice.

• Eat oily fish at least four times a week.

• Eat a tablespoon of ground sunflower, sesame, pumpkin, and linseeds, and live yogurt daily.

• Avoid "rich" and refined foods.

• Avoid mixing concentrated starches and concentrated proteins at the same meal.

• Try Aloe vera juice, which is available in health food stores and is drunk diluted with water, or Slippery Elm tea for their soothing properties.

BROWN RICE

• High in vitamins B1, B2, B3, B5, B6, E, and folic acid, and minerals chromium, magnesium, manganese, molybdenum, phosphorus, potassium, selenium, and silicon – for general health

ABOVE *Brown rice is delicious as well as very healthy and easy to digest.*

• Contains tocotrienols – antioxidants – for reducing cholesterol and preventing oxidative damage of digestive tract

• Contains phytochemicals to boost immune system and balance hormones

• No digestive inhibitors (often found in grains and beans) – easily digested

• Soluble fiber – healthy elimination of toxins

BELOW *Oily fish should be eaten four times a week.*

• Short chain fatty acids – heal the gut lining and prevent growth of toxic bacteria

ABOVE *Live yogurt is the one dairy food that can be freely consumed.*

LIVE YOGURT

• Lactose reduced (microbially changed to lactic acid) – little chance of allergic reaction

• Lactic acid – helps absorption of calcium and phosphorus

• Helpful bacteria – to rebalance gut flora

• High levels of calcium – for bones and teeth, and for calming nerves

ALOE VERA

• Contains mucopolysaccharides – good for fighting gut infections and candidiasis

• Contains balanced amino acids, enzymes, essential fatty acids, and mineral electrolytes – for general health

BELOW *Aloe vera may be prickly on the outside but it has many soothing properties.*

• Contains substances which reduce inflammation and help with lubrication – useful for soothing the digestive tract and arthritic conditions

• Contains substances which promote healthy cell growth after damage – useful for healing the digestive tract and for the skin

• Contains substances which help detoxify the liver and colon, thereby helping with elimination of wastes – good for constipation

• Contains substances which help with gall bladder function

• Contains substances which help promote a healthy cardiovascular system

• Contains substances which help asthma sufferers

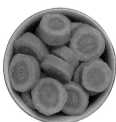

ABOVE *Carrots are best eaten raw.*

CARROTS (RAW)

• Beta-carotene – produces vitamin A – for intestinal lining integrity, and antioxidant activity

• Phytochemicals – immune stimulating

• Fiber – for healthy elimination

• Fructose – a "low glycemic" sugar; helps blood sugar balance

REMOVING FOOD INTOLERANCE

This program attempts to remove all common allergens. If you possess an intolerance to these allergenic foods, you will generally see an improvement within two to three weeks, after which you can reintroduce them one at a time and observe symptoms.

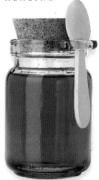

LEFT *Maple syrup can be used sparingly instead of sugar.*

- Avoid wheat, rye, corn, oats, and barley. Use brown rice, millet, and buckwheat, or any products made with these (e.g., rice noodles, buckwheat flour).

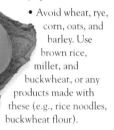

ABOVE *Eggs are avoided in this program.*

- Avoid dairy produce, and eggs. Use soy milk, soy cream, soy cheese, soy yogurt, rice milk.

- Avoid foods containing yeast (e.g., yeast extract spreads, bread, vinegar, and other fermented products).

- Avoid citrus fruits (orange, grapefruit, lemon, lime).

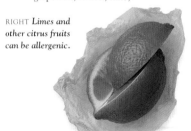

RIGHT *Limes and other citrus fruits can be allergic.*

- Avoid ordinary sugar and its products. Use honey, maple syrup, or fructose sparingly.

- Avoid all food additives. Use only fresh (not packaged) food.

- Avoid any foods to which you know you are allergic.

- Try a little vitamin C powder (1–3g daily) to help strengthen the system.

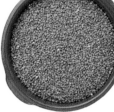

ABOVE *Non-allergenic buckwheat lacks gluten.*

BUCKWHEAT

- Lacks gluten – non allergenic

- High in B vitamins, and minerals magnesium and molybdenum – for general health

- Bioflavonoid (rutin) – prevention of free-radical damage

- Fiber – good elimination of toxins

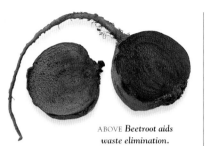

ABOVE **Beetroot aids
waste elimination.**

BEETROOT

• Excellent "blood-builder" due to its iron content

• A natural source of vitamins (especially vitamin C) and minerals (especially calcium, phosphorus, and iron) – for general health

• Highly alkali-forming – useful in helping remove acidity

• Bioflavonoid (anthocyanidin) – prevention of free-radical damage

• Fructose – "low-glycemic" sugar to help blood sugar balance

• Aids elimination of wastes and supports detoxification processes

ALFALFA SPROUTS

• Rich in nearly every vitamin and mineral, particularly boron (for strong bones) – for general health

• Good source of a wide range of amino acids – for healthy cell growth

• Contain phytochemicals and natural enzymes – to help prevent oxidative damage, promote digestive function, and remove toxins

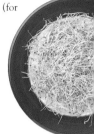

ABOVE **Alfalfa
sprouts contain
most vitamins.**

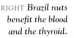

ABOVE **Walnuts
are good for the
skin and brain.**

WALNUTS

• Contain high levels of most B vitamins, especially B6; choline and inositol, vitamin E, calcium, potassium, manganese, and iron – excellent for nerve function and blood system

• Good balance of omega 6 and omega 3 essential fatty acids – excellent for the cardiovascular system, healthy skin, immune function, brain function, and hormones

BRAZIL NUTS

• High levels of many vitamins and minerals, especially copper – good for the blood

• Contain good levels of selenium, an antioxidant which protects against free radicals; this mineral also helps thyroid activity

RIGHT **Brazil nuts
benefit the blood
and the thyroid.**

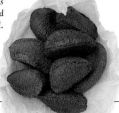

DETOXIFYING THE SYSTEM

This program attempts to encourage the removal of toxins, both from the tissues and the gut. It can be used for three to five days each month, or for one day every week.

- Eat only boiled brown rice, millet, and buckwheat (no other grains).

- Eat a wide range of vegetables (beetroot, broccoli, cabbage, carrots, cauliflower, celery, chicory, cress, lettuce, onions, garlic, leeks, potatoes, sweet peppers, sprouted alfalfa, and other sprouted seeds). Eat a good 60 percent of these raw.

- Eat plenty of fruit.

- Eat one tablespoon of seeds (sunflower, pumpkin, sesame, and linseed) per day.

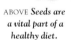

ABOVE *Seeds are a vital part of a healthy diet.*

- Eat a small amount of pulses (legumes), around 2oz (54g) per day, as the main protein food. One or two nuts can be eaten as well.

- Eat a very small amount of lean meat or fish; no more than 1oz (27g) per day.

LEFT *Detoxifying diets allow one or two nuts a day.*

- Omit all dairy foods, soy products, sugar, alcohol, tea, coffee, soft drinks, cordials, etc. Rice milk can be used.

- Drink around three to four pints (two liters) of filtered or bottled water per day.

RAW VEGETABLES (ESPECIALLY DARK-GREEN TYPES)

- High alkalinity – to offset acidity; extremely useful in detoxification

- Natural enzymes – to help digestion and elimination of toxins

- High in antioxidants and phytochemicals – protection against free-radical damage, immune stimulating, and hormone balancing

- Helpful for removing toxins from tissues into the blood for eventual elimination

- High in many vitamins (especially A, C, E, and K), and minerals (especially calcium and potassium), and bioflavonoids – excellent for general health

ABOVE *Drinking plenty of filtered water will flush out toxins.*

BELOW *Dark-green vegetables contain enzymes that aid digestion.*

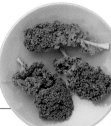

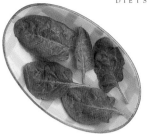

ABOVE *Eat spinach raw for maximum benefit.*

HEALING THE EFFECTS OF STRESS

This program cannot remove the causes of stress, but can help to optimize the diet so that there are sufficient body reserves to help combat its effects. It can be used indefinitely.

• Eat vegetables, fruits, and other foods containing antioxidants and phytochemicals.

• Avoid all refined, burnt, barbecued, and fried food.

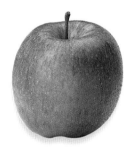

ABOVE *Apples are rich in antioxidants and pectin.*

• Do not overeat. Have five or six small meals every day to maintain blood sugar levels.

• Take a high quality multivitamin/multimineral supplement containing all essential nutrients but in particular the B vitamin group and vitamin C.

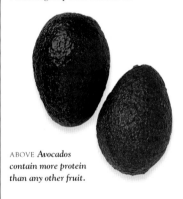

ABOVE *Avocados contain more protein than any other fruit.*

AVOCADO

• Excellent source of potassium – needed in high concentrations daily to heal the effects of stress.

• Good balance of omega 6 and omega 3 oils – for hormonal balance.

SIBERIAN GINSENG

• Ginseng is an excellent addition to any supplement regime as it helps to counteract the effects of stress.

BELOW *Ginseng tea is useful in stressful conditions.*

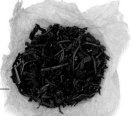

IMPROVING ATHLETIC PERFORMANCE

This program is for all those who undertake strenuous exercise frequently. It attempts to replace those nutrients lost in sweat and supply the body with extra nutrients required for energy production and muscle repair.

• Eat vegetables, fruits, and other foods containing antioxidants and phytochemicals.

• Eat at least one tablespoon of linseeds, sesame, and pumpkin seeds daily.

ABOVE *Strenuous exercise and training require a special dietary program.*

• Eat liver (unless pregnant or breastfeeding), or extra dark-green vegetables, twice a week, as well as other high protein foods.

• Have olive oil and wheatgerm daily.

• Take molasses regularly.

• Take a high quality multivitamin/multimineral supplement.

RIGHT *Linseeds contain mucins that protect the digestive tract.*

OLIVE OIL

• Good levels of vitamin E – antioxidant; also helps to "thin" the blood and keeps the cardiovascular system working well

• Copper – useful for formation of blood cells, and as a coenzyme

• Monounsaturated fatty acids – help to keep circulation system healthy and in the prevention of heart disease

• Contains oleuropein – helps to lower blood pressure

MOLASSES

• High in vitamins and minerals – an excellent food for general health

LINSEEDS (FLAXSEED)

• High in vitamins and minerals – for general health

• Omega 3 fatty acids – for immune system, hormonal balance, healthy skin and muscles

• Whole linseeds – excellent for curing and preventing constipation

• Contain mucins – for coating and protecting the digestive tract

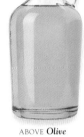

ABOVE *Olive oil helps to keep the cardiovascular system working well.*

OPTIMIZING CARDIOVASCULAR HEALTH

This program attempts to encourage a healthy heart, clear arteries and veins, reduce cholesterol, and improve circulation.

• Take soy milk, soy cheese, soy yogurt, rice milk, and oat milk instead of dairy products.

• Eat oily fish in preference to meat.

• Eat plenty of dark-green and orange vegetables and fruits.

• Eat vegetables from the onion family, especially garlic

• Take one tablespoon of ground mixed seeds (especially linseed) daily.

• Keep saturated fats and refined carbohydrates to an absolute minimum.

• Avoid all foods containing hydrogenated fats or trans fatty acids.

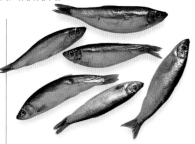

ABOVE *In oily fish the oil is found throughout the flesh, not just in the liver as in white fish.*

GARLIC

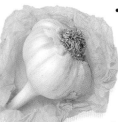

ABOVE *Garlic helps cleanse the blood and reduce blood pressure.*

• Sulfur – for cleansing the blood

• Selenium – antioxidant – for preventing free-radical damage

• Germanium – for generating energy, helping lower cholesterol and blood pressure

• Excellent for heart and circulation, in part due to its concentration of bioflavonoids and phytochemicals

• A natural antibiotic and antifungal food

OILY FISH

• EHA and DHA – essential fatty acids – immune stimulating, balancing hormones, healthy skin, membranes, and cardiovascular health

• Protein – excellent quality

• Calcium – for strong bones and teeth, and the nervous system

• Excellent source of vitamins and minerals – good for energy production, nervous system, brain function, and thyroid function

GINKGO BILOBA

• Contains antioxidants and phytochemicals which help improve blood flow and cerebral metabolism, and protect against oxidative damage

KEEPING BONES AND CONNECTIVE TISSUE HEALTHY

This program will help alleviate some of the symptoms of arthritic conditions and will also help improve bone density.

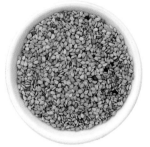

ABOVE *Sesame seeds are high in B and E vitamins as well as the mineral calcium.*

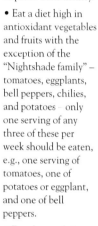

ABOVE *Good dietary habits help improve bone density.*

• Eat a diet high in antioxidant vegetables and fruits with the exception of the "Nightshade family" – tomatoes, eggplants, bell peppers, chilies, and potatoes – only one serving of any three of these per week should be eaten, e.g., one serving of tomatoes, one of potatoes or eggplant, and one of bell peppers.

• Eat plenty of oily fish and ground mixed seeds, especially sesame and linseed.

• Eat dairy foods sparingly; replace with soy products and/or rice milk.

• Limit red meat and foods containing saturated fat, hydrogenated fat, trans fatty acids, or processed fats.

RIGHT *Arthritic conditions can be aggravated by wheat.*

• Avoid common food allergens (e.g., wheat).

• Supplement the diet with fish oils and other anti-inflammatory nutrients.

SESAME SEEDS

• High in B vitamins – for healthy nerves and energy production

• Good levels of vitamin E – for a healthy cardiovascular system

• Good levels of calcium, magnesium, and phosphorus – for strong bones and teeth

• Contains manganese and zinc – for healthy cells

• Omega 6 fatty acids – for immune system, hormonal balance, and healthy skin

• Contains sesamin – to help reduce the amount of serum and liver cholesterol

• Sesame oil – to help protect against colon cancer

IMPROVING HORMONE BALANCE

This program will help to alleviate some of the symptoms of PMS, menstruation, and the menopause.

• Eat a large proportion of your vegetables raw.

• Choose vegetables and fruits packed with antioxidants and phytochemicals.

• Eat one tablespoon of ground mixed seeds daily.

• Eat fish, poultry, and tofu as main proteins.

• Avoid saturated fats, red meat, alcohol, and processed foods.

• Eat five or six small meals a day, each a good balance of carbohydrate and protein.

• Insure the diet contains plenty of soybeans and soy products.

• Take a high quality multivitamin/multimineral supplement and Evening Primrose oil capsules daily.

ABOVE *Mangoes are exceptionally high in beta-carotene, which the body converts to Vitamin A.*

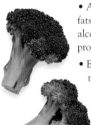

ABOVE *There is some evidence that broccoli contains anticancer compounds.*

SOY AND ITS PRODUCTS

This information applies to all soy products except texturized soy.

• Phyto-estrogens – to help rebalance sex hormones; useful in PMS, menopause

• Protein – excellent protein (tofu), especially for vegetarians

• Phytochemicals – to help immune function and hormonal system

• Good levels of vitamins (especially B6, B12, biotin), choline, and inositol – for healthy nerve and brain function, and energy production

• Good levels of vitamin E – for healthy cardiovascular function and alleviating PMS breast tenderness

• Good levels of calcium, magnesium, and boron – for strong bones and teeth, and the nervous system

• Contains potassium – helps heart function

• Soy Lecithin Granules – for helping reduce cholesterol and in weight reduction

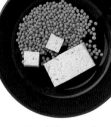

ABOVE *Soybeans and tofu are important for improving the hormone balance.*

PREVENTING INFECTION AND FATIGUE

This program attempts to improve the disease-fighting capability of the immune system, and reduce fatigue.

• Choose your vegetables, fruits, and other foods from the lists on pages 41, 42, and 43. Vegetables and fruits containing vitamin C are immune stimulating and cleansing.

• Eat food from an organic source wherever possible.

• Eat vegetables from the onion family frequently.

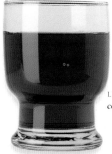

ABOVE *The onion family helps prevent fatigue.*

• Eat at least one tablespoon of ground mixed seeds, especially pumpkin seeds, daily.

• Drink elderberry cordial.

LEFT *Elderberry cordial is widely available in health food stores.*

• Have very few wholegrain carbohydrates, and no refined types whatsoever.

• Avoid dairy foods and saturated, hydrogenated, or processed fats; use soy milk, soy cheese, soy yogurt, rice milk, lean meats, and fish.

• Avoid stimulant drinks.

• Supplements of vitamin C (1–3g per day), beta-carotene, zinc, and shiitake extract may be helpful.

ORGANIC PRODUCE

• Reduces level of pollutants in diet

• Usually higher in range of vitamins, minerals, antioxidants, and phytochemicals, than non-organic produce

PUMPKIN SEEDS

• High in many minerals (especially zinc) – excellent for immune system, reproductive system, wound healing, skin health, brain function

ABOVE *Pumpkin seeds are good for several body systems and the skin.*

• Omega 3 fatty acids – immune stimulating, hormonal balance, skin health

• Contains good levels of the B vitamins, folic acid, and vitamin E – for healthy nerves and circulatory system.

LOSING WEIGHT

You will find that after several weeks on the New Pyramid program your weight will begin to normalize without you having to consciously try to "reduce weight." The following can also be tried to help the process.

• Insure you limit your food intake to the portion sizes and suggested food ratios as given on pages 32 and 33.

• Consume slow release carbohydrates, such as fibrous vegetables, oats, and millet.

• Eat a daily quota of seeds, especially linseeds. Fenugreek seeds or fenugreek tea are useful for balancing blood sugar level.

• Spread your foods throughout the day in five or six small meals, but try not to eat after 8.00pm; insure each small meal is well balanced for protein and carbohydrate, as suggested on pages 32 and 33.

• Avoid drinking any alcohol on an empty stomach, since this will only encourage you to eat more at the next meal.

• Avoid all refined and convenience foods.

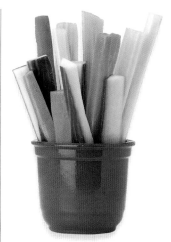

ABOVE *Raw vegetable sticks are the healthy way to cure hunger pangs.*

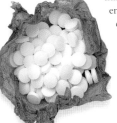

ABOVE *Zinc is an important trace element in our diet.*

• If you feel hungry at any time, make a drink of diluted apple juice and water (1:1 ratio), and add $\frac{1}{2}$ teaspoon of fructose, and $\frac{1}{4}$ teaspoon vitamin C powder.

• If you need something "solid" to snack on, have a bowl of crudités (raw sticks of carrot, celery, cucumber, or other vegetables) and a few pumpkin seeds.

• Take a daily high quality multivitamin/multimineral supplement, which supplies good levels of all the essential vitamins and minerals, especially the B vitamins, magnesium, zinc, selenium, and iodine.

FOODS TO HELP YOU MAINTAIN WEIGHT LOSS

The following foods are particularly good for accelerating weight loss.

SEAWEED

Seaweed means sea vegetables such as kelp and nori.

• An excellent source of minerals, especially iodine (for thyroid function), iron, calcium, magnesium, cobalt, and silicon

• An excellent source of vitamin B complex, D, E, and K – for general health

• Contains many phytochemicals – to help immune and hormonal function

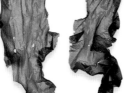

ABOVE *Seaweed is rich in iodine – vital for thyroid function.*

WHEATGERM

ABOVE *Wheatgerm is particularly beneficial during childbearing years.*

• Very good levels of the B vitamins, folic acid (excellent source for women in childbearing years), biotin, and the mineral iron – for increasing energy levels

• Good amounts of vitamin E – for circulation and hormone balance

• Contains choline and inositol – for fat metabolism and helping reduce cholesterol

• Good levels of minerals magnesium, phosphorus, zinc, manganese, and molybdenum – for general health

GARCINIA CAMBOGIA

Extract of the plant Garcinia Cambogia (grown in South East Asia) is available in freeze-dried capsules sold in healthfood stores.

• A rich source of hydroxy-citrate, which is thought to be involved in the metabolism of fats and cholesterol, and helps to increase the rate of fat-burning – has been found to be useful in weight reduction diets.

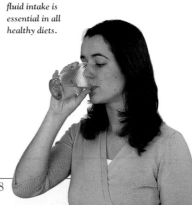

BELOW *Adequate fluid intake is essential in all healthy diets.*

Further reading

THE NEW BOOK OF FOOD COMBINING:
by *Jan Dries* (Element Books, 1995)

200 NEW FOOD COMBINING RECIPES
by *Inge Dries* (Element Books, 1995)

FATS THAT HEAL, FATS THAT KILL: by
Udo Erasmus (Alive Books, 1993)

HEALING THROUGH NUTRITION
by *Dr. Melvyn R Werbach*
(HarperCollins, 1995)

LIVING FOOD – THE KEY TO HEALTH
& VITALITY by *Patrick Holford*
(ION Press, 1996)

VITAMINS & MINERALS: A STEP-BY-
STEP GUIDE by *Karen Sullivan*
(Element Books, 1997)

THE COMPLETE ILLUSTRATED GUIDE
TO NUTRITIONAL HEALING by *Denise
Mortimore* (Element Books, 1998)

Useful addresses

**American Academy of
Environmental Medicine**
4510 W.89th Street, Prairie Village
Kansas 66207, USA

American College of Nutrition
722 Robert E Lee Drive, Wilmington
NC20927, USA

**American Preventive
Medical Association**
275 Millway, PO Box 732, Barnstable
ME 02630, USA

**Institute for Optimum Nutrition
(ION)**
Blades Court, Deodar Road, London
SW15 2NU, England

**The Society for Promotion
of Nutritional Therapy (SPNT)**
PO Box 47, Heathfield, East Sussex
TN21 8ZX, England

**The Soil Association
(for Organic Suppliers in the UK)**
40–56 Victoria Street, Bristol
BS1 6BY, England

**Australian College of Nutritional
& Environmental Medicine**
13 Hilton Street, Beaumaris
Victoria 3193, Australia

**Australian Natural Therapists
Association**
Taren Point, PO Box 2517
Sydney 2232, Australia

Association of Natural Therapies
81 Forest Hill Road, Milford
Auckland, New Zealand

**Society for
Orthomolecular Medicine**
16 Florence Avenue, Toronto
Canada, M2N1E9